Branka Strazisar

Postoperative pain treatment after breast cancer surgery

Branka Strazisar

Postoperative pain treatment after breast cancer surgery

LAP LAMBERT Academic Publishing

Impressum / Imprint
Bibliografische Information der Deutschen Nationalbibliothek: Die Deutsche Nationalbibliothek verzeichnet diese Publikation in der Deutschen Nationalbibliografie; detaillierte bibliografische Daten sind im Internet über http://dnb.d-nb.de abrufbar.
Alle in diesem Buch genannten Marken und Produktnamen unterliegen warenzeichen-, marken- oder patentrechtlichem Schutz bzw. sind Warenzeichen oder eingetragene Warenzeichen der jeweiligen Inhaber. Die Wiedergabe von Marken, Produktnamen, Gebrauchsnamen, Handelsnamen, Warenbezeichnungen u.s.w. in diesem Werk berechtigt auch ohne besondere Kennzeichnung nicht zu der Annahme, dass solche Namen im Sinne der Warenzeichen- und Markenschutzgesetzgebung als frei zu betrachten wären und daher von jedermann benutzt werden dürften.

Bibliographic information published by the Deutsche Nationalbibliothek: The Deutsche Nationalbibliothek lists this publication in the Deutsche Nationalbibliografie; detailed bibliographic data are available in the Internet at http://dnb.d-nb.de.
Any brand names and product names mentioned in this book are subject to trademark, brand or patent protection and are trademarks or registered trademarks of their respective holders. The use of brand names, product names, common names, trade names, product descriptions etc. even without a particular marking in this work is in no way to be construed to mean that such names may be regarded as unrestricted in respect of trademark and brand protection legislation and could thus be used by anyone.

Coverbild / Cover image: www.ingimage.com

Verlag / Publisher:
LAP LAMBERT Academic Publishing
ist ein Imprint der / is a trademark of
OmniScriptum GmbH & Co. KG
Heinrich-Böcking-Str. 6-8, 66121 Saarbrücken, Deutschland / Germany
Email: info@lap-publishing.com

Herstellung: siehe letzte Seite /
Printed at: see last page
ISBN: 978-3-659-77275-7

Zugl. / Approved by: Ljubljana, Univeristy of Ljubljana, Diss., 2014

Copyright © 2015 OmniScriptum GmbH & Co. KG
Alle Rechte vorbehalten. / All rights reserved. Saarbrücken 2015

Branka Stražišar, dr. med.

A COMPARISON OF LOCAL AND SYSTEMIC POSTOPERATIVE PAIN TREATMENT AFTER BREAST CANCER SURGERY

I dedicate this thesis to my dearest ones: Kristina, Matej and Sara, my husband Borut and my mother

ACKNOWLEDGMENTS

I would like to thank my mentor, prof. dr. Nikola Bešić, for all his expert help with the completion of this thesis and encouragement during all creative blocks.

I would like to thank the members of the Commission – prof. dr. Mark Snoj, prof. dr. Mojca Kržan and prof. dr. Mirt Kamenik for all their remarks and advice that helped improve this thesis.

I would like to thank all the patients for their participation.

I would like to thank the surgical oncologists and the plastic surgeons for the key work in the study.

I would like to thank the doctors and nurses at the Institute of Oncology in Ljubljana who have helped me with the work. I would especially like to thank Nurse Irma Mrzelj and the nurses from Analgesia for their reliable help with the collection of data. I wish to thank Nurse Margareta Gradišek for her eager recording of the first data after surgery. I would also like to thank all other co-workers at the Oncological Institute who have helped me conduct this study.

I would like to thank mag. Mateja Blas for performing the statistical analysis and all the useful guidance. I also wish to thank doc. dr. Vesna Zadnik for the additional help with statistics.

And finally, I would also like to thank the Management of the Institute of Oncology, which has – despite the economic crisis – enabled me to complete my doctoral degree.

TABLE OF CONTENTS

1 INTRODUCTION 11
   1.1 The Significance of Acute Postoperative Pain Treatment 11
   1.2 Pain after Breast Cancer Surgery 13
   1.3 Methods for Relieving Acute Pain after Breast Cancer Surgery 15
   1.4 Benefits of Using Local Anaesthetics for Pain Treatment in Cancer Patients 16
   1.5 Relieving Pain after Breast Cancer Surgery at the Institute of Oncology 17
   1.6 An Overview of the Data on the Use of Local Anaesthetics in the surgical wound 18
      1.6.1 Oncological Breast Cancer Surgery 18
      1.6.2 Reconstructive Breast Surgery 20
      1.6.3 A Summary of the Conducted Randomized Studies 24

2 PURPOSE OF THE STUDY, WORKING HYPOTHESIS AND SPECIFIC GOALS 26
   2.1 Working hypothesis 26
   2.2 Specific goals 26

3 PATIENTS AND METHODS 27
   3.1 Description of the examinees 27
   3.2 Design of the study 30
      3.2.1 Detailed description of the study 30
   3.1 Pain Measurement 32
   3.2 Assessment of Alertness 33
   3.3 Nausea, Vomiting and Medication Consumption 33
   3.4 Complications after Surgery 33
   3.5 Chronic Pain 33
   3.6 Statistical Analysis 34

4 RESULTS 35
   4.1 Acute Pain 38
      4.1.1 Axillary Dissection Patients 38
      4.1.2 Patients after Immediate Reconstruction with a Tissue Expander 40
   4.1 Consumption of Opioids and Other Analgesics, Alertness 42

	4.1	Postoperative Nausea 44
	4.2	Complications 45
	4.3	Hospitalization 45
	4.4	Late Complications 45
5	DISCUSSION 46
6	CONCLUSIONS 51
7	SOURCES AND LITERATURE 52

TABLES, GRAPHS, FIGURES AND APPENDIX

Table 1: Patient characteristic (first group of examinees – after axillary lymph node dissection) 28

Table 2: Patient characteristic (second group of examinees – after immediate reconstruction) 29

Table 3: Patient treatment, adjuvant treatment, hospitalization and complications (first group of examinees – after axillary dissection) 36

Table 4: Patient treatment, adjuvant treatment, hospitalization and complications (second group of examinees – after immediate reconstruction) 37

Table 5: Pain intensity (first group of examinees – after axillary dissection) 38

Table 6: Pain intensity (second group of examinees – after immediate reconstruction) 40

Table 7: Drug consumption and alertness (first group of examinees – after axillary dissection) 43

Table 8: Drug consumption and alertness (second group of examinees – after immediate reconstruction) 43

Graph 1: VAS at rest (left) and on movement (right) in the recovery room, on the day of surgery and on the first potoperative day (first group of examinees – after axillary dissection) 39

Graph 2: VAS at rest (left) and on movement (right) in the recovery room, on the day of surgery and on the first potoperative day (second group of examinees – after immediate reconstruction) 41

Graph 3: Piritramide consumption in the first 24 postoperative hours 44

Graph 4: Metoclopramide consumption in the first 24 postoperative hours 44

Figure 1: Structure of the study (first group of examinees – after axillary lymph node dissection) 30

Figure 2: Structure of the study (second group of examinees – after immediate reconstruction) 31

Appendix 1: DN4 Questionnaire 54

LIST OF ABBREVIATIONS

APS	acute pain service
ASA	American Society for Anaesthesiology
BMI	body mass index
EGF	endothelial growth factor
IASP	International Association for the Study of Pain
OAA/S	observer's assessment of alertness/sedation scale
PCA	patient controlled analgesia
PONV	postoperative nausea and/or vomiting
SNB	sentinel node biopsy
VAS	visual analogue scale

I. ABSTRACT

A Comparison of Local and Systemic Pain Treatment after Breast Cancer Surgery

<u>Background:</u> Perioperative analgesia has traditionally been provided by opioid analgesics, which have many adverse effects. The efficacy of local anaesthetics after breast cancer surgical procedures has already been studied, but there is no satisfactory scientific proof of the advantage of local anaesthetics in comparison to systemic opioid pain treatment.

Our aim was to find out if pain treatment with an elastomeric pump with a local anaesthetic is more effective in breast cancer patients after surgical procedures than systemic pain treatment.

The specific aims of our study were to find out if patients treated with an elastomeric pump with a local anaesthetic have

1. less acute pain at rest or on movement of an upper limb immediately after surgery and during the first days after surgery,

2. less opioid consumption during the first days after surgery and experience less adverse effects of opioids (sedation, respiratory depression, nausea, vomiting),

3. less chronic pain three months after operation

in comparison to patients treated with systemic pain treatment.

<u>Materials and methods:</u> We prospectively randomized 120 patients undergoing a surgical procedure for breast cancer. Half of the patients had undergone axillary dissection, while the other half had breast cancer surgery with immediate breast reconstruction with a tissue expander. The patients included were surgically treated at the Institute of Oncology in Ljubljana from December 2010 to May 2012. A written consent for the participation in the study was obtained from all of the patients.

The test subgroup was treated with continuous local anaesthetic applied by a wound catheter, while the other subgroup was treated with standard intravenous analgesia.

Data on postoperative pain at rest and on movement of the upper limb was collected every three hours on the day of surgery and then every eight hours during hospitalization. The consumption of piritramide was recorded. The alertness of patients six hours after the surgical procedure was estimated by using the observer's assessment of alertness/sedation scale (OAA/S Scale). Nausea and use of antiemetic were recorded.

The presence of chronic pain was established three months after immediate reconstruction with a tissue expander. After axillary lymphadenectomy, the presence of chronic neuropathic pain, oedema of the arm and reduction of shoulder mobility was established after six months.

Results: Patients treated with an elastomeric pump with a local anaesthetic had significantly less acute pain immediately after the surgical procedure than patients treated with systemic pain treatment. Patients treated with an elastomeric pump with a local anaesthetic consumed significantly less piritramide in the first 24 hours after surgery. Consequently, they experienced fewer adverse effects of opioids, they were more alert six hours after surgery and they needed less antiemetic drugs than patients treated with systemic pain treatment. The proportion of patients who were treated with an elastomeric pump with a local anaesthetic and had chronic pain was smaller in comparison to patients treated with systemic treatment.

Conclusion: The use of an elastomeric pump with a local anaesthetic is an effective, safe, patient- and staff-friendly method for postoperative pain relief in breast cancer patients after axillary dissection and after primary breast reconstruction with a tissue expander. The use of continuous infusion of a local anaesthetic into the surgical wound reduces acute pain immediately after the surgical procedure and also on the day of surgery. It is an effective method of postoperative pain treatment without adverse effects. It enables smaller opioid consumption in the first 24 hours after the surgical procedure and higher alertness and does not cause postoperative nausea. Patients treated with a local anaesthetic have a lower frequency of chronic pain three months after the surgical procedure compared to patients treated with standard analgesia.

Key words: breast cancer, postoperative pain, elastomeric pump, wound catheters, local anaesthetic, piritramide

1 INTRODUCTION

1.1 The Significance of Acute Postoperative Pain Treatment

Pain is defined by the IASP (International Association for the Study of Pain) as an unpleasant sensory and emotional experience associated with actual or potential tissue damage (1).

The purpose of postoperative pain treatment is to provide comfort to patients and improve the results of surgery. We wish to suppress the autonomic and somatic reflexes, which are triggered by nociceptive impulses activated by surgical injury (2). Reducing postoperative stress is one of the most important goals of patient care. We want to preserve the patient's natural resistance, which has been lowered due to surgical injury, general anaesthesia and treatment with opioids (3). The purpose of postoperative pain treatment is to stimulate the restoration of organ functions, enable the patient to breathe, cough, move and eat normally and thereby recuperate as quickly as possible (2).

The first acute pain service (APS) was established in the USA and in Germany in 1985 with the aim of improving postoperative pain treatment. This was soon followed by a quick expansion of services with the use of specialized methods for pain treatment in hospitals of the developed countries. The following methods were established: patient-controlled analgesia (PCA), infusions of opioid analgesics and local anaesthetics into the epidural space and surgical wounds. Pain treatment with specialized methods has contributed to improving patient well-being and reduced respiratory complications. But questions such as are the mentioned methods effective enough, what are the adverse effects, do patients tolerate them well, what is the effect on hospitalization and the costs of treatment, remain open. A comprehensive paper has shown a significant reduction of postoperative pain with the use of APS (4). The most common adverse effects of the methods themselves were: postoperative nausea and/or vomiting (PONV), urine retention and sedation (4).

Pain causes stimulation of nociceptors, nerve inflammation or nerve injury in neuropathic pain. Effective treatment of postoperative pain is also important for the prevention of development of chronic pain. The transition to chronic pain depends on numerous factors: genetic design, past experience with pain, psychological effects and age. If we knew how to determine the risk of chronic pain, we could act preventively with more intensive and longer analgesia in predisposed patients (5).

The surgical procedure and the inflammation that follows stimulate the receptors for pain in the skin – nociceptors. The pain stimulus is transmitted through A delta fibres and thin C fibres to the central nervous system. As they enter the spinal cord, primary neurons connect to secondary projection neurons. Some secondary neurons have synaptic connections to local interneurons prior to connection (6). At the spinal cord level, it is possible to inhibit the pain stimulus by transmitting impulses from wide dynamic range neurons – gate control theory. Wide dynamic range neurons transmit impulses of thicker fibres – A beta and pain impulses. An impulse from A beta fibres can suppress pain impulses through interneurons in the spinal cord. Descending inhibition or excitation of pain neurons at the spinal cord level is also possible (7). Secondary projection neurons pass through to the other side of the spinal cord and conduct information to supraspinal structures (6). The phylogenetically older pathway is more medial – posterior fascicle, which consists of the paleospinothalamic, spinoreticular, spinomesencephalic, spinoparabrachial-amygdaloidic, spinoparabrachial-hypothalamic and spinohypothalamic bundle (7). Slower pain is transmitted via an older pathway, stimulation goes mostly out of C fibres. The localization of slow pain is imprecise (8). The phylogenetically younger pathway leads across the anterolateral fascicle, which consists of the neospinothalamic bundle, the spinocervical bundle and the polysynaptic bundle of the dorsal horn of the spinal cord (7). The localisation of fast pain is good, particularly if the tactile receptors, which are conducted through the medial lemniscus, are also stimulated (8). The main structure of sensory information, reception, integration and transmission of potential is the thalamus with its numerous nuclei (9). As in the spinal cord, there are numerous interactions between neurons with possible inhibition in the thalamus (6). Tertiary neurons spread from the thalamus to the cerebral cortex to three areas: to the primary somatosensory cortex, to the secondary somatosensory cortex and to the frontal cingulate cortex (10). The efferent filaments from the thalamic nuclei and subcortical areas are divided into two parallel, complementary systems – the lateral and medial system, similarly as the afferent filaments from the spinal cord to the cortex and the brainstem, which are divided into the medial and lateral part. The older medial system mostly ends before the thalamus in the brainstem (8). The perception of learning and memory also goes to the primary and secondary somatosensory cortex and joins the perception of pain (11). Emotional information and memory of painful experience also go to the limbic cortex and frontal cingulate cortex and intertwine with pain information (7). The brain itself suppresses pain signals with the endogenous analgesic system. The most known nuclei are *locus ceruleus*, which secretes noradrenalin, and *nucleus raphe* in the brainstem, which secretes serotonin (6). The hypothalamus and epiphysis secrete beta-endorphins. Approximately twelve substances similar to opiates can be found in various parts of the brain (8). Postoperative pain is an unavoidable consequence of stimulated pain receptors, while the perception of the feeling itself is very complex.

1.2 Pain after Breast Cancer Surgery

Sensitivity of the breast area travels through intercostal nerves, which are the branches of the anterior spinal nerves. The pectoralis major and the pectoralis minor muscle innerve *n. pectoralis medialis* and *lateralis*, both are spinal, primarily motor nerves, which arise from the brachial plexus, while some of the filaments arise also from the first thoracic segment. Deep sensitivity, perception of movement, pressure, proprioception of the thoracic area is conducted via spinal nerves from C5 to Th1 (12).

Sufficient postoperative pain relief is becoming increasingly important in the treatment of cancer patients (13). The feeling of pain is an individual experience, which depends on previous experience and the patient's current state (14). Anxiety before a surgical procedure is a risk factor for greater postoperative pain (15). Patients who come to hospital for planned breast cancer surgery are worried due to the nature of the disease and the still unclear further treatment. Their distress is reflected also in postoperative pain. The memory of pain that has been experienced in the past and in which a cognitive process is involved is important for the feeling of current pain (16). Based on what has been stated above, it can be concluded that coping with one's diagnosis and the patient's past experience of pain affects the perception of postoperative pain after breast cancer surgery.

Among various operations for breast cancer, the most severe pain is present after axillary lymph node dissection and breast reconstruction with a tissue expander (17). Despite precise surgical technique, sensory nerve fibres of intercostobrachial nerves can be injured during axillary dissection (18). The intercostobrachial nerve originates from the second or sometimes third intercostal nerve and continues into the lateral cutaneous branch, innerves the medial and the posterior part of the upper arms, joins the medial brachial cutaneous nerve. The third intercostal nerve often has its own large lateral cutaneous branch, which represents the second intercostobrachial nerve (12). Even a small injury to the nerve can already cause pain (18). Intercostal nerves are mixed – motor and sensory. Two important motor nerves pass through the axilla – *n. thoracicus longus* and *n. toracodorsalis*, which the surgeon locates and preserves during the preparation of the axilla. Injury to these two nerves causes muscle deficit and deformation of posture (19). Injury to *n. thoracicus longus* causes loss of innervation of *m.seratus anterior* and winged scapula (*scapula alata*). Injury to *n. thoracicus longus* is very unpleasant, but rare, because it can be avoided by through surgical preparation. *N. toracodorsalis* innerves *m. latissimus dorsi*. Injury to *n. toracodorsalis* causes reduced medial rotation and adduction of the arm (12). Axillary lymph node dissection for breast cancer can cause: pain, feeling of numbness of the skin, paresthesia, muscle weakening and lymphoedema. Temporary pain, numbness of the skin or paraesthesia occur in 35 – 50 % of the patients despite good surgical technique (19). As much as 30 % of patients develop chronic pain (19). Occurrence of chronic pain is often a consequence of inadequately treated acute pain (20,21).

More and more patients want breast reconstruction after mastectomy. At the Breast Unit of the Humanitas Centre in Milan[1], patients decided in favour of reconstruction after mastectomy in 82 percent of the cases (22). For patients with small, minimally ptotic breasts, tissue expander or an implant is an appropriate method of reconstruction. The benefits of this method are: simple surgical procedure, no injury due to removal of patient's own tissue, the structure of the material used is similar to breast tissue, quick operation, quick recovery after procedure (23). But despite the simplicity of the operation, severe pain is present afterwards, which is not adequately reduced after opioids (17). Severe pain after implant insertion is frequent

---

[1] Breast Unit, Humanitas Cancer Center, Milano.

also after aesthetic breast augmentation surgery with implants (24). Pain relief has not been adequate after these procedures despite large doses of opioids (17,24).

Mechanosensitive pain receptors, from which signals are conducted via thin myelinated A delta fibres or unmyelinated C fibres, are present in the muscles (25).

Pain after breast reconstruction with a tissue expander is the most severe postoperative pain among all the operations for breast cancer and often leads to chronic pain (17). The stretching of skin simulates nociceptors in the skin, while the stretching of muscles stimulates mechanosensitive pain receptors in the muscles (25). Occurrence of chronic pain is more likely because the pain is severe (20). It is not yet completely clear whether acute pain causes the occurrence of chronic pain. The mechanisms of the occurrence of chronic pain are the consequence of several factors and are complex. Continuous stimulation of nociceptors can cause chronic pain. The duration and intensity of the initial injury leads both to peripheral and central hypersensitivity, which together affect the perception of pain (26).

1.3 Methods for Relieving Acute Pain after Breast Cancer Surgery

Opioid analgesics are traditionally used for postoperative analgesia. Large systemic doses of opioids cause several adverse effects: depression of breathing, dizziness, drowsiness, postoperative nausea and vomiting, itchiness of the skin, urine retention, ileus, constipation (27). Long-term use of opioids can lead to psychological or physical addiction (28).

In order to avoid the adverse effects of opioids as much as possible, anaesthesiologists and surgeons are increasingly using non-opioid techniques of pain treatment in the perioperative period (29). Continuous infusion of local anaesthetics into the surgical wound for postoperative analgesia has proven itself as an effective anti-pain treatment in a meta-analysis of studies with randomised patients (30). Local anaesthetics can improve postoperative pain treatment (26). Local anaesthetics inhibit afferent nociceptive signals and the inflammatory reaction (31).

A local anaesthetic is used to interrupt the conduction of nerve impulses, which are created with the stimulation of skin and muscle nociceptors, and interrupt the conduction via intercostal nerves. The local anaesthetic blocks the transmission of nerve impulse by inhibiting the penetration of sodium ions through the nerve cell membrane. The conduction through thin C pain fibres and thicker A delta fibres is interrupted. Based on their structure, local anaesthetics are divided into ester and amide anaesthetics (32). The long-acting amide local anaesthetics, which are most commonly used for pain management after surgery, are: ropivacaine, bupivacaine and levobupivacaine.

Levobupivacaine is a long-acting amide local anaesthetic and analgesic. It inhibits nerve conduction in sensory and motor nerves, primarily by acting on voltage-sensitive sodium channels on the cell membrane, but it also acts on potassium and calcium channels. Moreover, levobupivacaine can hinder the transfer and transmission of impulses in other tissue, whereby the effects on the brain and the cardio-vascular system as well as the central nervous system are the most important for the occurrence of adverse effects, which nevertheless rarely occur (from $\geq 1/10,000$ to $<1/1,000$) (33).

1.4 Benefits of Using Local Anaesthetics for Pain Treatment in Cancer Patients

The use of local anaesthetics instead of opioids is particularly beneficial in patients with cancer patients. The surgical procedure and general anaesthesia suppress immunity after surgery (3,34). Opioids also suppress immunity (3,35,36). Local anaesthetics reduce the need for opioids and thereby contribute to reduced immunosuppression (3). Gupta *et al.* established that morphine stimulates tumour angiogenesis and growth of breast tumour xenograft via G protein receptors in mice (34). The situation is reversed with local anaesthetics. Sakaguchi *et al.* have proven on tongue cancer cell culture that lidocaine has a direct inhibitory effect on the epidermal growth factor (EGF) and directly inhibits cell proliferation (37). Exadaktylos *et al.* found fewer recurrences of breast cancer after continuous infusion of local anaesthetics into the paravertebral space than with intravenous opioid PCA during the initial years of follow-up (38). Biki *et al.* found in a follow-up period of 2.8 to 12.8 years a reduced risk of biochemical recurrence of prostate cancer with the use of epidural anaesthesia and continuous postoperative epidural analgesia in combination with general anaesthesia in comparison to only general anaesthesia and intravenous opioid PCA analgesia (3). Merquiol *et al.* found less recurrences of laryngeal and hypopharynx cancer after cervical epidural anaesthesia and analgesia than with intravenous opioid analgesia (39).

Local anaesthetics for the treatment of postoperative pain are used in several fields of surgery. Studies with the use of local anaesthetics in the wound have been conducted in the field of orthopaedic, abdominal, gynaecological, urologic, cardiothoracic and breast and axillary surgery (40).

1.5 Relieving Pain after Breast Cancer Surgery at the Institute of Oncology

At the Institute of Oncology, we use piritramide, an opioid analgesic under the trade name Diplodor, for standard anti-pain treatment after breast cancer surgery. Piritramide is a synthetic opioid. Analgesic action of piritramide is somewhat weaker than of morphine, it has 65 – 75 % of analgesic action of morphine. Among the opioids, piritramide is very suitable for the use in the postoperative period, because it causes less respiratory arrests and nausea than other opioids (41,42). Aside from an opioid analgesic, we also use metamizole (Analgin), a non-opioid analgesic, in intravenous form on the day of surgery at the Institute of Oncology. We have good experience with intravenous analgesia itself in terms of pain prevention. But we are not satisfied with the occurrence of adverse effects. Drowsiness, nausea, and vomiting are often very unpleasant. Patients are inactive when using opioids. If patients did not have pain and nausea, they could move more after surgery.

From the first postoperative day on we treat pain with non-opioid analgesics *per os*: paracetamol, alone or in combination with tramadol (Zaldiar, Doreta), a medium-strength opioid, and non-steroidal analgesics, most often diklofenakom (Olfen, Naklofen).

At the Institute of Oncology, we began using an infusion of a local anaesthetic into the surgical wound, which is administered by catheter and elastomeric pump, in October 2008. We used levobupivacaine (Chirocaine 0.25 %). At the end of surgery we injected a single dose of local anaesthetic by catheter. Despite the initial dose of a local anaesthetic we noticed that we had to add also an opioid and metamizole before the end of surgery, so that patients did not have pain at waking. We reported on our experience with elastomeric self-deflating pumps with a local anaesthetic at the

XXIX. Annual Congress of the European Society of Regional Anaesthesia and Pain Therapy in 2010 (43). We established that a local aesthetic, injected into the wound, effectively reduces pain after axillary dissection for breast cancer surgery, and enables significantly lower consumption of the opioid drug piritramide. In patients with associated diseases, hospitalization was shorter after the application of a local anaesthetic than in patients who did not receive a local anaesthetic. We did not record any inflammation or other complications after the use of a catheter for analgesia (43).

1.6 An Overview of the Data on the Use of Local Anaesthetics in the surgical wound

1.6.1   Oncological Breast Cancer Surgery

Five studies on the use of local anaesthetics in the surgical wound have been published in the field of surgical treatment of axillary and breast cancer. One study is retrospective and was conducted by Jacobs and Morrison (13). They included 41 patients after breast cancer surgery or with carcinoma *in situ*. Before the end of the surgical procedure they inserted two drains 2-3 cm apart into the surgical wound and connected them to an elastomeric pump with 270 ml of a local anaesthetic for analgesia after surgery. The catheters were inserted 3-5 cm below the wound. They were placed on the lateral side of the mastectomy wound and were not stitched. The catheters were fenestrated 6.5 cm in length. 0.25 % bupivakain with adrenaline was used, flow rate in each catheter was two ml/hour. They established reduced postoperative pain, whereby opioid consumption was reduced by 2/3. The other four studies on the use of local anaesthetics in the surgical wound were prospective randomized. Schell (19) included 27 patients who had undergone axillary lymph node dissection for breast cancer in his study. The patients were randomized into three groups. The test group was treated with a wound catheter connected to an elastomeric pump with 0.5 % bupivacaine, a local anaesthetic, the placebo group also had a catheter inserted, but the pump contained saline solution, while the standard group received oral opioid analgesics. The catheters for analgesia were perforated 10 cm in length. The catheter was inserted after completed axillary lymph node dissection under the axillary vein and secured with a stitch. The catheter was inserted into the mid axillary line, above the exit site of the suction drains. Pump flow rate was 0.5 ml/hour, volume was 60 ml, continuing for five days. The group receiving bupivacaine had less pain during all five days, less opioid consumption, they experienced less drowsiness and had less antiemetics consumption. The results of the study indicate the efficacy of a local anaesthetic, but the number of patients was too small to prove the efficacy of the use of local anaesthetics in the surgical wound for the treatment of postoperative pain.

Talbot *et al.* published a study on the use of a local anaesthetic, injected into the surgical wound by an axillary drain (44). 42 patients after mastectomy for breast cancer were included in the study. The patients were randomized into a test and a control group, which received a placebo. The test group received 20 ml of 0.5 % bupivacaine every four hours six times, the control group received saline solution. The drains were clamped for 20 minutes after each injection. Both groups received morphine intravenously via a pump, which was controlled by the patient herself (PCA). The study did not show differences between the two groups regarding morphine consumption. Pain was measured with the visual analogue scale (VAS) and the score was low in both groups; there was no statistically significant difference.

Fassoulaki *et al.* published a study on the use of a local anaesthetic in the surgical wound along with the use of other drugs (45). A local anaesthetic was injected only at the end of surgery, drains were not inserted. 50 patients with breast cancer were included in the study and randomized into a test and a placebo group. The test group received a skin cream with a local anaesthetic – EMLA, in the morning before surgery and three days afterwards, gabapentine tablets already before surgery and also eight days postoperatively, and at the end of surgery the surgeon injected 10 ml of 0.75 % ropivacaine into the brachial plexus area and 3 ml of 0.75 % ropivacaine into the 3rd, 4th and 5th intercostal space. The placebo group received saline solution instead of a local anaesthetic, cream without a local anaesthetic and placebo tablets. Analgesics consumption after surgery was lower in the test group. After three and after six months, the test group had less chronic pain. The multimodal approach has proven itself effective for the treatment of postoperative pain. But it is not clear to what extent each of the three methods of treatment helps prevent pain.

Sidiropoulou *et al.* randomized patients and compared continuous infusion of a local anaesthetic in the surgical wound and a single-injection paravertebral block (46). 48 patients were included in the study; the procedure performed was modified radical mastectomy. Half of the patients received 20 ml of 0.5 % ropivacaine into the paravertebral space at the level of the third thoracic vertebra before general anaesthesia. The other half of the patients had two perforated catheters inserted in the axilla and above the pectoralis major muscle by a surgeon. They immediately started with the application of 0.5 % ropivacaine with a flow rate of 2 ml/hour to each side for 24 hours. Both catheters were connected to an elastomeric pump. After four hours, pain was lower in the group with a paravertebral block than in the group with a catheter. Arm movement was better and less painful. But after 16 and 24 hours, pain was lower in the group with a catheter and arm movement was less restricted. There were no differences in opioid consumption between the two groups. But more nausea was observed in the group with a catheter. Continuous wound infiltration of a local anaesthetic has proven itself as an effective alternative to paravertebral anaesthesia.

1.6.2 Reconstructive Breast Surgery

The number of studies published so far is low also in the field of reconstructive breast surgery. We found only one prospective randomized study after delayed breast reconstruction. Prospective studies after immediate breast reconstruction were not found, but two retrospective studies after immediate reconstruction were found. A few more studies have been conducted after cosmetic breast augmentation, six studies were found (24,47-51).

1.6.2.1 Studies after Breast Augmentation For Cosmetic Reasons

We found six published studies on the use of local anaesthetics in the surgical wound after breast surgery for cosmetic reasons (24,47-51). Three of these were conducted with the use of a wound catheter and three with a single injection of a local anaesthetic at the end of surgery.

1.6.2.2 Studies with Wound Catheters after Cosmetic Breast Augmentation

Rawal *et al.* (24) randomized 60 patients into a test and a standard group. Patients in the test group applied a local anaesthetic themselves as PCA. They used 10 ml of 0.25 % ropivacaine for the left breast and 10 ml of 0.5 % ropivacaine for the right breast. The standard group received tablets, 1 g of paracetamol four times a day and

500 mg of ibuprofen three times a day. Pain was lower in the group of patients with regional analgesia, postoperative opioid consumption was lower, antiemetics consumption was lower and patient satisfaction was greater than in the group of patients treated with standard analgesia. The catheter was placed subcutaneously, perforated and inserted through an incision wound along the entire length of the breast. The catheter had an anti-bacterial filter. It was connected to a 100 ml elastomeric pump.

Pacik established the benefits of continuous infusion of a local anaesthetic versus single injection in patients after breast augmentation surgery with implants (50). He included 41 patients, all of whom received continuous infusion of a local anaesthetic into one breast and two methods of injection of a single dose (10 or 20 ml of 0.25 % bupivacaine every 4 or 6 hours) with a syringe into the other breast. Both methods have proven themselves as effective, some patients supported the continuous method considering the pain experienced, while others supported single doses. Interestingly, the finding was made that after injection of a local anaesthetic into one breast, pain reduced in both breasts in 42 % of patients. Narcotics consumption was reduced after the use of a local anaesthetic. The price of continuous infusion is higher because of the self-deflating pump (the price was $200).

Kazmier *et al.* investigated the efficacy of a continuous infusion of 0.5 % bupivacaine in the surgical wound in comparison to a continuous infusion of saline solution in the wound in patients after cosmetic breast augmentation with implants in a prospective, randomised, double-blind study. The side of injection of a local anaesthetic was unknown and was determined with random inclusion. Patients daily rated the average intensity of pain on each side at home. Pain on the side of injection of a local anaesthetic was lower the first four days, but it did not reach statistical significance. The conclusion of the study is that a continuous infusion of bupivacaine means a trend towards less postoperative pain (51). They wanted to avoid different pain evaluation in different patients in the study. But the downsides of this study are that the number of patients included was small, the patients completed the questionnaire at home and the patients were restrained by the pump. The infusion flow rate and dispersion across the entire surface of the wound were perhaps also not optimal.

1.6.2.3 Studies after Breast Augmentation with a Single Application of a Local Anaesthetic

We found three studies with a single injection of a local anaesthetic into the surgical wound site (47-49). The test groups were compared to the placebo group. Mahabir *et al.* published the results of a study on the control of postoperative pain in 100 patients after breast augmentation surgery in 2004 (47). One hundred patients were divided into 4 groups. Into the implant pocket they applied: 1) 15 ml of saline solution (control group, which received the placebo); 2) 30 mg of ketorolac; 3) 150 mg of bupivacaine with adrenaline or 4) 150 mg of bupivacaine with adrenaline, together with 30 mg of ketorolac. The group with bupivacaine and ketorolac had the least pain after surgery and spent the least amount of time in the recovery room.

In 2008, Mahabir *et al.* published the findings of the second part of the study on pain in 50 patients after breast augmentation surgery with implants, where pain was observed during the first ten postoperative days (48). Patients were randomized into the test group, in which 150 mg of bupivacaine with adrenaline together with 30 mg of ketorolac were placed into the implant pocket, and to the control group, which received only saline solution. Pain and codeine consumption were measured during the first 10 days after surgery. The group, which received bupivacaine and ketorolac, had a significantly lower intensity of pain, it had less codeine consumption. The results of both studies have shown that postoperative pain was lower in patients who received local anaesthetics than in the control group.

McCarty *et al.* conducted a randomized prospective study on the effect of injecting 0.5 % bupivacaine, a local anaesthetic, into the implant pocket on postoperative pain (49). Fifty patients after reconstruction with implants were randomized into two groups, one group received a local anaesthetic applied into both implant pockets, the other group did not receive anything. Neither the patients nor the nurses in the recovery room knew which patient received a local anaesthetic and which did not. The patients in the test group had 15 ml of solution injected into the implant pocket on each side, 0.5 % bupivacaine 15 ml (=75 mg), and ketorolac – 30 mg in 15 ml of saline solution. VAS was significantly lower during the first three postoperative hours after drug injection in comparison to those patients who did not receive drugs. After six hours postoperatively there were no more differences in pain between the two groups. Opioid consumption was higher in the test group during the first three postoperative days. This was probably due to the unexpected occurrence of pain, when the local anaesthetic stopped acting. Pain was lower in the test group immediately after surgery, but when the local anaesthetic stopped acting, pain reoccurred. This is probably the reason why consumption of opioid medicinal products was higher in the control group during the first three postoperative days, but there were no differences in opioid consumption between the two groups on the fourth to fifth postoperative day.

1.6.2.4 Study after Delayed Breast Reconstruction

Legeby *et al.* conducted a study on pain using a local anaesthetic applied to the surgical wound by catheter for analgesia in patients after delayed reconstruction with implants who had been previously operated for breast cancer (52). 43 patients were included and randomized into the test and the placebo group. In all of the patients, a surgeon infiltrated the skin with a local anaesthetic with adrenaline before incision. All patients had an epidural catheter inserted into the implant pocket before the wound was closed. The test group received 15 ml of 0.25 % levobupivacaine every three hours, while the placebo group received saline solution. Injection was repeated fifteen times and then stopped approximately 45 hours after surgery. All patients received intravenous PCA with an opioid. All of them also received paracetamole. If reduction mammaplasty was performed on the other breast at the same time, a catheter was inserted also on that side and 10 ml of 0.25 % levobupivacaine was injected before wound closure, followed by 10 ml of 0.2 % ropivacaine every three hours. The test group, which received levobupivacaine, had significantly less pain according to VAS during the first 15 postoperative hours. Pain was lower on movement the first 6 hours after operation and again for the interval 18 – 24 hours in the levobupivacaine group. Opioid consumption was lower in the levobupivacaine group, but the difference was not significant.

1.6.2.5 Studies after Immediate Breast Reconstruction with a Tissue Expander

We found two studies with local anaesthetics after immediate breast reconstruction with a tissue expander, the comparator group was retrospective in both of them. Lu *et al.* included patients after reduction mammaplasty and after mastectomy with immediate reconstruction with a tissue expander (53). One part of the patients was the standard retrospective control group – 39 patients times two, while the test group consisted of 35 patients times two, who received 0.25 % bupivacaine, a local anaesthetic, by wound catheter with a flow rate of 2 ml/hour. Epidural catheters were used. The patients in the test group with a local anaesthetic had significantly less pain in the recovery room than the standard retrospective control group. Since the patients were discharged very quickly, it was not possible to observe them for a longer period. The patients who were treated with a local anaesthetic in the wound and who underwent only reductional mammaplasty were hospitalized for a distinctly shorter time than the control standard group, because they were mostly discharged from hospital already on the day of surgery. A trend towards shorter hospitalization was noticeable also after immediate reconstruction, only there was no statistically significant difference.

Turan *et al.* conducted a study in a similar manner with a control standard retrospective group in patients after breast cancer surgery with immediate reconstruction (54). 60 patients were included altogether; one half was the retrospective control group, while the other 30 patients received single doses of 10 - 15 ml of 0.2 % ropivacaine by wound catheter. Epidural catheters were used. Opioid consumption was significantly lower in the group with a local anaesthetic.

1.6.3 A Summary of the Conducted Randomized Studies

In none of the studies had it been stated that complications with the wound occurred because of the use of catheters: wound infection, delayed wound healing or haematoma (13,19,24,31,44,47-54). The published results even show infection is impeded with the use of local anaesthetics (55).

The impeding effect on wound healing has been proven by inhibition of protein synthesis on cell culture through inhibition of the G protein receptor (56). A clinically significant effect on wound healing has not been recorded in any of the studies with local anaesthetics in the wound (13,19,24,31,44,47-54). Ropivacaine and levobupivacaine have the least impeding effect on wound healing (56).

In the studies listed above, systemic adverse effects of local anaesthetics were not recorded. There is very little possibility of the anaesthetic passing directly into a blood vessel, because the surgeon inserts the wound catheter for analgesia under visual control. Continuous application of a drug prevents sudden increases in blood concentration, and single doses are small and far from toxic doses. The toxic dose is highest with ropivacaine, followed by levobupivacaine, which is the next safest local anaesthetic (57).

Studies on the use of local anaesthetics in the surgical wound after breast cancer surgery included a small number of patients (between 27 and 100), which is why the patient groups were small. Rawal, Lu and Turan compared the test group with standard treatment (24,53,54). Other authors used a placebo group for comparison (19,31,44,47,48,51) or nothing (a form of placebo), as McCarty *et al.* had done (49), or they compared two methods of injecting a local anaesthetic (46,50). Differences in VAS for measuring pain were greater in the studies with a test group, which was using a placebo, in comparison with the studies that had a control group with standard analgesia.

Pacik compared two methods of application of the same drug (50). Talbot *et al.* (44) found little pain in his study, because all of the patients – regardless of the group – also had an intravenous pump with opioids for PCA. Local anaesthetics reduced pain more effectively than the placebo in all of the studies (19,24,31,47,48,51,52). An exception was the study conducted by Talbot *et al.*, where there were no differences in the intensity of pain between the two groups after application of a local anaesthetic (44). The reason for this is probably that Talbot did not use fenestrated catheters, and the suction drains did not enable dispersion of the local anaesthetic across the wider surface of the wound (44). Based on that we conclude that the position of the wound catheter is significant, as well as the extent of wound coverage with a local anaesthetic. Local anaesthetics were more effective than standard treatment also in the studies with a standard control group.

Our good experience regarding postoperative analgesia with an elastomeric pump and a local anaesthetic does not yet mean that this method of pain treatment is more effective than standard systemic analgesia. In order to prove that, we have conducted a prospective randomized study.

2 PURPOSE OF THE STUDY, WORKING HYPOTHESIS AND SPECIFIC GOALS

The purpose of the study is to confirm the hypothesis on reducing pain after breast cancer surgery with the use of a local anaesthetic, which is applied to the wound by a catheter connected to a self-deflating pump, with a prospective, randomized study.

2.1 Working hypothesis

We assume that patients after breast cancer surgery who were treated with local anaesthetics, which are applied to the wound by a catheter connected to an elastomeric self-deflating pump, experience less pain than patients who were treated only with systemic analgesics.

2.2 Specific goals

With the doctor's thesis we wish to examine, whether:

1. patients after axillary node dissection for breast cancer who will be treated with a local anaesthetic will experience less pain than patients treated only with systemic analgesics.

2. patients after immediate breast reconstruction with a tissue expander who will be treated with a local anaesthetic will experience less pain than patients treated only with systemic analgesics.

3. patients after axillary node dissection for breast cancer who will be treated with a local anaesthetic will require less opioids and antiemetics and will be more alert than patients treated only with systemic analgesics.

4. patients after immediate breast reconstruction with a tissue expander who will be treated with a local anaesthetic will require less opioids and antiemetics and will be more alert than patients treated only with systemic analgesics.

5. chronic pain will occur less often in patients after axillary node dissection for breast cancer treated with a local anaesthetic than in patients treated only with systemic analgesics.

6. chronic pain will occur less often in patients after immediate breast reconstruction with a tissue expander treated with a local anaesthetic than in patients treated only with systemic analgesics.

3 PATIENTS AND METHODS

3.1 Description of the examinees

We presented the study to the patients who came to the Institute of Oncology for breast cancer surgery with axillary lymph node dissection and the patients who wanted immediate reconstruction after breast cancer surgery and requested their written consent for participation in the study.

Before anaesthesia, patients were examined according to our standard procedure. This includes basic information on body build, the presence of concomitant diseases, the presence of allergies and habits, use of medication and an evaluation of the anaestesiological risk according to ASA (American Society of Anaesthesiology). We collected data on the presence of pain before surgery and the use of analgesics.

The parameter for inclusion was axillary lymph node dissection for breast cancer or breast cancer surgery with immediate reconstruction with implants. Parameters for exclusion were allergies to local anaesthetic or piritramide, male gender, pregnancy and high risk because of anaesthesia, ASA score above 3, age lower than 18 years. The characteristics of the first group of examinees are presented in Table 1, the characteristics of the second group of examinees are presented in Table 2.

Republic of Slovenia National Medical Ethics Committee approved the study on 16th November 2010 with Decision Nr. 22pk/12/10 on 11/24-2010.

Table 1: Patient characteristic (first group of examinees – after axillary lymph node dissection)

Characteristic		Group with a local anaesthetic*	Standard group*	Value p
Number of patients		30	30	-
Age (years)		57.4 (13)	62.9 (12)	0.79
Height (m)		1.62 (0.07)	1.637 (0.06)	0.43
Weight (kg)		72.7 (12.7)	73.8 (16.4)	0.76
Body mass index (kg/m^2)		27.68 (5.3)	27.43 (5.2)	0.86
ASA scale	1	7 (23 %)	3 (10 %)	0.46
	2	22 (73 %)	25 (83 %)	
	3	1 (3 %)	2 (7 %)	
Concomitant diseases		19 (63 %)	24 (80 %)	0.25
Diabetes		4	8	0.33
Fibromyalgia		0	1	-
Rheumatoid arthritis		0	0	-
Depression		1	4	0.35
Side with cancer	Left	18 (60 %)	20 (67 %)	0.79
	Right	12 (40 %)	10 (33 %)	
Type of invasive carcinoma	Ductal	28 (93 %)	27 (90 %)	1.00
	Lobular	2 (7 %)	3 (10 %)	
Tumour diameter (cm)		2.66 (0.1-15.0)	2.43 (0.5-6.0)	0.57
Grade	I	0 (0 %)	1 (3 %)	1.00
	II	11 (37 %)	11 (37 %)	
	III	19 (63 %)	18 (60 %)	
Metastatic lymph nodes		5.2 (0-34)	5.3 (0-24)	0.37
Dissected lymph nodes		17.3 (5-34)	19.3 (8-28)	0.15
Positive hormone receptors		24 (82.8 %)	26 (86.7 %)	0.73
HER-2 positive		5 (16.7 %)	6 (20 %)	1.00

*Numerical variables in the parentheses are listed as an average value (SD) or median (range); for descriptive variables, numbers are listed (%)

Table 2: Patient characteristic (second group of examinees – after immediate reconstruction)

Characteristic		Group with a local anaesthetic*	Standard group*	Value p
Number of patients		30	30	-
Age (years)		47.6 (9)	48.0 (9)	0.88
Height (m)		1.66 (0.07)	1.66 (0.05)	0.78
Weight (kg)		60.9 (8.6)	62.5 (11.8)	0.56
Body mass index (kg/m^2)		22.2 (2.9)	22.6 (4.4)	0.61
ASA scale	1	10 (33 %)	15 (50 %)	0.44
	2	19 (63 %)	14 (47 %)	
	3	1 (3 %)	1 (3 %)	
Concomitant diseases		15 (50 %)	14 (47 %)	1.0
Diabetes		0	0	-
Fibromyalgia		0	0	-
Rheumatoid arthritis		0	0	-
Depression		3	1	0.61
Side of mastectomy	Left	7 (23 %)	15 (50 %)	0.10
	Right	15 (50 %)	10 (33 %)	
	Bilateral	8 (27 %)	5 (17 %)	
Type of invasive carcinoma (N=60)	Invasive ductal carcinoma	22 (73 %)	17 (57 %)	0.56
	Invasive lobular carcinoma	2 (7 %)	2 (7 %)	
	Ductal *in situ*	1 (3 %)	2 (7 %)	
	Without carcinoma	5 (17 %)	9 (30 %)	
Tumour diameter (cm)		1.2 (0-5)	1.3 (0-6.5)	0.76
Grade (N=58)	0	5 (17 %)	9 (31 %)	0.66
	I	2 (7 %)	1 (3 %)	
	II	11 (38 %)	9 (31 %)	
	III	11 (38 %)	10 (35 %)	
Metastatic lymph nodes – median and range		0 (0-21)	0 (0-18)	0.98
Dissected lymph nodes – median and range		2 (0-33)	3 (0-27)	0.97
Positive hormone receptors		18 (60 %)	20 (67 %)	0.79
HER-2 positive		5 (17 %)	7 (23 %)	0.75

*Numerical variables in the parentheses are listed as an average value (SD) or median (range); for descriptive variables, numbers are listed (%)

3.2 Design of the study

It is a prospective randomized clinical study on the effect of two methods of pain treatment on pain intensity. Our hypothesis was that the method of postoperative pain treatment affects pain intensity (VAS), wakefulness after surgery (observer's alertness/sedation scale, intravenous opioid consumption (mg of piritramide), postoperative nausea– we measured antiemetics consumption, chronic pain occurrence (questionnaire). Patients did not undergo any additional invasive procedures due to the study.

3.2.1 Detailed description of the study

There were two groups of examinees. The first group of examinees consisted of 60 patients after breast cancer surgery with axillary lymph node dissection (Figure 1), while the other group consisted of 60 patients after mastectomy and immediate reconstruction with a tissue expander (Figure 2). Patients were randomized into two groups after signing the consent for participation in the study. Randomization was performed by the Research Unit of the Institute of Oncology. A filled out protocol on fulfilment of the criteria for inclusion was sent to the Research Unit for each patient and was then sent back by the Research Unit, stating whether a patient was placed in the test group or the standard (control) group.

STUDY DESIGN

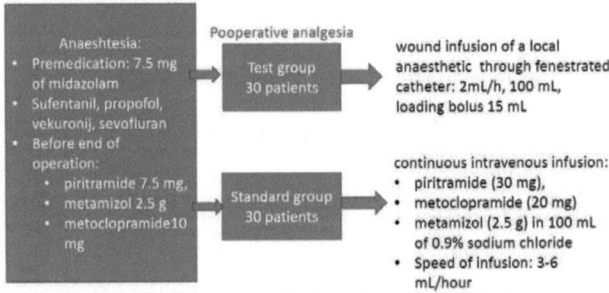

Figure 1: Structure of the study (first group of examinees – after axillary lymph node dissection)

- January 2011 – April 2012
- Randomization – Unit for clinical research

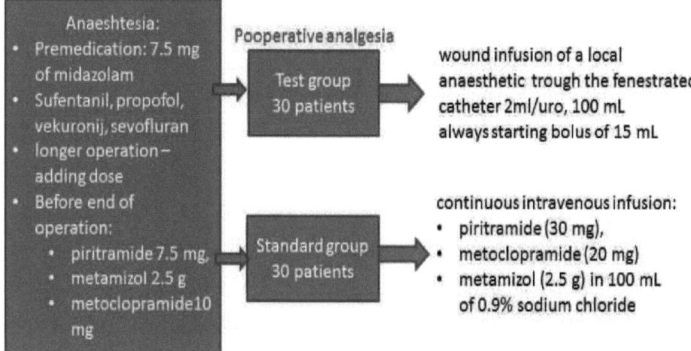

Rescue dose for both groups: piritramide 3 mg iv, metoclopramide 10 mg iv

Figure 2: Structure of the study (second group of examinees – after immediate reconstruction)

Anaesthesia was performed in the same way in all patients. Patients received a premedicational tablet - 7.5 mg of midazolam at the ward one hour before the operation. After brief ventilation with oxygen, we began anaesthesia with sufentanil 0.1μg/kg, propofol 2 mg/kg and vecuronium 0.08 mg/kg. After orotracheal intubation, patients were artificially ventilated with 40 % O_2 and 60 % N_2O with an adjustment to the exhaled pressure of CO_2 between 3.9 – 4.5 kPa. Anaesthesia was maintained with sevoflurane in a concentration of 1.5 vol % and sufentanil 0,1 μg/kg in a single dose before surgical incision and in the second group of examinees again before the beginning of reconstruction. The second group of examinees was also given a single dose of vecuronium in a dose of 0.02 mg/kg before the beginning of reconstruction. After completed surgery, the neuromuscular block was reversed, if necessary, with 1 mg of atropine and 2.5 mg of neostigmine. All four subgroups received piritramide, (Dipidolor) 7.5 mg, metamizole (Analgin) 2.5 g and metoclopramide (Reglan) 10 mg intravenously before surgery was completed.

The surgical procedure was performed by experienced oncological and plastic surgeons, 11 oncological surgeons participated in the axillary dissection, and 10 oncological surgeons and 9 plastic surgeons in primary reconstruction. The method of work was comparable in all of them.

Patients, who were randomized into the comparator standard subgroup, were given piritramide (30 mg), metoclopramide (20 mg) and metamizole (2.5 g) in 100 ml of saline solution by continuous intravenous infusion on the day of surgery. The nurses at the ward set the infusion flow rate between 3 - 6 ml/hour, or to the lowest flow rate which still ensured adequate analgesia. Both patient groups received a saving dose of 3 mg of piritramide intravenously in case of pain, and an antiemetic (metoclopramide 10 mg) in case of nausea. Patients who were randomized into the test group received a local anaesthetic for pain by wound catheter connected to an elastomeric pump. 0.25 % levobupivacaine was used in the test group, the patients received a single dose of 15 ml of 0.25 % levobupivacaine (37.5 mg) immediately after the procedure. Surgical drains were clamped for five minutes in order for the single dose to spread throughout the wound. After five minutes, we opened the catheter, which was connected to an elastomeric pump with 100 ml (250 mg) of 0.25 % levobupivacaine. Flow rate was 2 ml/hour. The catheter was removed after two days. After axillary lymph node dissection, the surgeon placed the catheter for analgesia above the muscles along the entire length of the wound. The catheter was fenestrated 15 cm in length. After the operations with immediate reconstruction with a tissue expander, the catheter was placed under the pectoralis major muscle, so that the entire width of the wound was affected. The type of catheter was the same as in the operations without dissection, the catheter was fenestrated 15 cm in length. The catheter was placed in the upper part of the wound, the anaesthetic ran downwards the entire operated part.

3.1 Pain Measurement

Pain was measured by using the visual analogue scale (VAS) ranging from 0 to 10 at rest and at adduction of the arm. The first measurement was done in the recovery room, then every three hours on the day of surgery, and then every eight hours during hospitalization. In literature, reduced pain was observed with the use of local anaesthetics, pain was mostly reduced by 25 % according to VAS. Since each group consisted of 30 patients, this was a large enough number to establish differences in pain.

3.2 Assessment of Alertness

Alertness was assessed according to the observer's assessment of alertness/sedation scale (OAA/S) (58) 6 hours after surgery. The OAA/S comprises four categories: 1) reaction to call, 2) speech, 3) facial expressions, 4) eyes (openness, clarity). The scale ranges from 1 (deep sleep) to 5 (alert). The result is the lowest value, recorded by the observer – a nurse in any category.

3.3 Nausea, Vomiting and Medication Consumption

In case of nausea, patients were first given 10 mg of metoclopramide, and, if that was not effective, 1 mg of granisetron; if there was still no improvement, the patients received 1.25 mg of droperidol intravenously. We recorded the amount of used piritramide, metamizole and metoclopramide in the first 24 hours. All patients received analgesics in the form of tablets on the first postoperative day. They received 100 mg of diclofenac, a combination of tramadol and paracetamol and an antiemetic in case of nausea.

3.4 Complications after Surgery

We recorded all postoperative complications, where medical intervention was necessary: bleeding, drain leakage, hemodynamic instability. We recorded occurrences of inflammation of the postoperative wound.

3.5 Chronic Pain

Tri months postoperatively the patients were asked again whether chronic pain has occurred, patients after axillary lymph node dissection were examined after six months at the outpatient clinic for pain treatment and it was established based on the DN4 questionnaire whether they have chronic pain. The presence of lymphedema and arm mobility was examined. Chronic pain was not evaluated in the second group of examinees after six months, because the patients where operated again for insertion of a permanent implant at the time.

3.6 Statistical Analysis

Depending on data distribution, the Student's t-test or the Mann-Whitney U test was used. Relationships between categorical variables were tested with the hi^2 test or Fisher's exact test. All comparisons were two-sided. A p-value of < 0.05 was considered as statistically significant. Two statistical programs – PASW 18 (SPSS Inc., Chicago, IL, USA) and R2.11.1 (R Foundation for Statistical Computing, Vienna, Austria) – were used.

4 RESULTS

The average age of the examinees in the first group (patients after axillary lymph node dissection) was 60 years (30–84), average height was 163 cm (150-176), average weight was 73 kg (43– 114), average body mass index (BMI) was 27.4 (15.4–41.4). There were no significant differences between the groups in either BMI, the score according to the American Society of Anaesthesiology (ASA) scale, concomitant diseases, patohistological characteristics of the tumour, number of dissected axillary lymph nodes (Table 1), type or length of operation, complications or hospitalization, the volume of seroma or the number of seroma punctures (Table 3).

Table 3: Patient treatment, adjuvant treatment, hospitalization and complications (first group of examinees – after axillary dissection)

		Group with a local anaesthetic*	Standard group*	Value p
Operation	Modified radical mastectomy	16 (53 %)	19 (63 %)	0.29
	Axillary dissection	13 (43 %)	8 (27 %)	
	Quadrantectomy with axillary dissection	1 (3 %)	3 (10 %)	
Length of operation (minutes)		72 (30-150)	62 (30-125)	0.18
Extent of axillary dissection	Three levels	29 (97 %)	28 (93 %)	0.61
	Two levels	1 (3 %)	2 (7 %)	
Number of patients with seroma puncture		19 (63 %)	23 (77 %)	0.42
Seroma – average volume per patient (ml)		206 (0-2040)	353 (0-1970)	0.24
Number of punctures due to seroma – average value		1.77 (0-10)	2.83 (0-14)	0.15
Neoadjuvant chemotherapy	Yes	6 (20 %)	4 (13 %)	0.73
	No	24 (80 %)	26 (87 %)	
Postoperative chemotherapy	Yes	22 (73 %)	18 (60 %)	0.21
	No	8 (27 %)	12 (40 %)	
Postoperative radiation	Yes	19 (63 %)	19 (63 %)	1.00
	No	11 (37 %)	11 (37 %)	
Hormone treatment	Yes	24 (80 %)	25 (83 %)	1.00
	No	6 (20 %)	5 (17 %)	
Hospitalization (days)		1.8 (1-7)	1.6 (2-5)	0.22
Haematoma		2 (6.7 %)	1 (3.3 %)	1.00
Operated again due to haemorrhage		2 (6.7 %)	1 (3.3 %)	1.00
Inflammation		5 (16.7%)	4 (13.3%)	1.00

*Numerical variables in the parentheses are listed as an average value (SD) or median (range); for descriptive variables, numbers are listed (%)

The average age of the examinees in the second group (patients after immediate reconstruction) was 47.8 years (25–64), lower than in the first group of examinees, average height in the second group of examinees was 166 cm (153-178), average weight was 61.7 kg (45– 85), average was BMI 22.4 (17–31.2). There were no significant differences between the patient subgroups of the second group of examinees in either BMI, the score according to the American Society of Anaesthesiology (ASA) scale, concomitant diseases, patohistological characteristics of the tumour, number of dissected axillary lymph nodes (Table 2), type or length of operation, complications or hospitalization (Table 4).

Table 4: Patient treatment, adjuvant treatment, hospitalization and complications (second group of examinees – after immediate reconstruction)

		Group with a local anaesthetic*	Standard group*	Value p
Operation on the breast (N=73)	Mastectomy; unilateral	23 (77 %)	24 (80 %)	0.58
	Mastectomy; bilateral	7 (23 %)	6 (20 %)	
Operation on the lymph nodes	Axillary dissection	6 (20 %)	5 (17 %)	1.00
	Biopsy of the sentinel lymph node; unilateral	21 (70 %)	22 (73 %)	1.00
	Biopsy of the sentinel lymph node; bilateral	3 (10 %)	3 (10 %)	
	No procedure on the lymph nodes	6 (20 %)	5 (17 %)	
Reconstruction	Tissue expander; unilateral	21 (70 %)	20 (67 %)	1.00
	Tissue expander; bilateral	9 (30 %)	10 (33 %)	
Length of operation - median (minutes)		140 (80-195)	120 (70-540)	0.62
Neoadjuvant chemotherapy	Yes	4 (13 %)	3 (10 %)	1.00
	No	26 (87 %)	27 (90 %)	
Postoperative chemotherapy	Yes	13 (43 %)	10 (33 %)	0.60
	No	17 (57 %)	20 (67 %)	
Postoperative radiation	Yes	9 (30 %)	3 (10 %)	0,11
	No	21 (70 %)	27 (90 %)	
Hormone treatment	Yes	17 (57 %)	19 (63 %)	0.79
	No	13 (43 %)	11 (37 %)	
Hospitalization (days)		5.2 (3-9)	5.4 (4-9)	0.61
Haematoma		2 (7 %)	1 (3 %)	1.00
Operated again due to haemorrhage		1 (3 %)	1 (3 %)	1.00
Inflammation		1 (3 %)	3 (10 %)	0.61

*Numerical variables in the parentheses are listed as an average value (SD) or median (range); for descriptive variables, numbers are listed (%)

4.1 Acute Pain

4.1.1 Axillary Dissection Patients

Graph 1 shows pain intensity after axillary lymph node dissection according to the VAS scale measured on movement and at rest in the recovery room, on the day of surgery and on the first postoperative day. Data on pain according to the VAS scale is presented in Table 5.

Table 5: Pain intensity (first group of examinees – after axillary dissection)

		Group with a local anaesthetic*	Standard group*	Value p
VAS** in the recovery room	on movement	0.0 (0-4)	1.0 (0-6)	<0.05
	at rest	1.0 (0-9)	3.0 (0-7)	<0.02
VAS on the day of surgery	on movement	0.3 (0-3.7)	1.5 (0-5.0)	<0.005
	at rest	1.3 (0-5.3)	3.2 (0-6.0)	<0.007
VAS first postoperative day	on movement	0.3 (0-3.3)	1.2 (0-4.0)	<0.05
	at rest	3.2 (1-5.7)	3.8 (0-6.0)	<0.119
Pain after three months (*number of patients*)		5 (17 %)	15 (50 %)	0.01
Pain after six months (*number of patients*)		6 (20 %)	12 (40 %)	0.09

*Numerical variables in the parentheses are listed as an average value (SD) or median (range); for descriptive variables, numbers are listed (%)

**VAS = visual analogue scale

Recovery room

On the day of surgery

First postoperative day

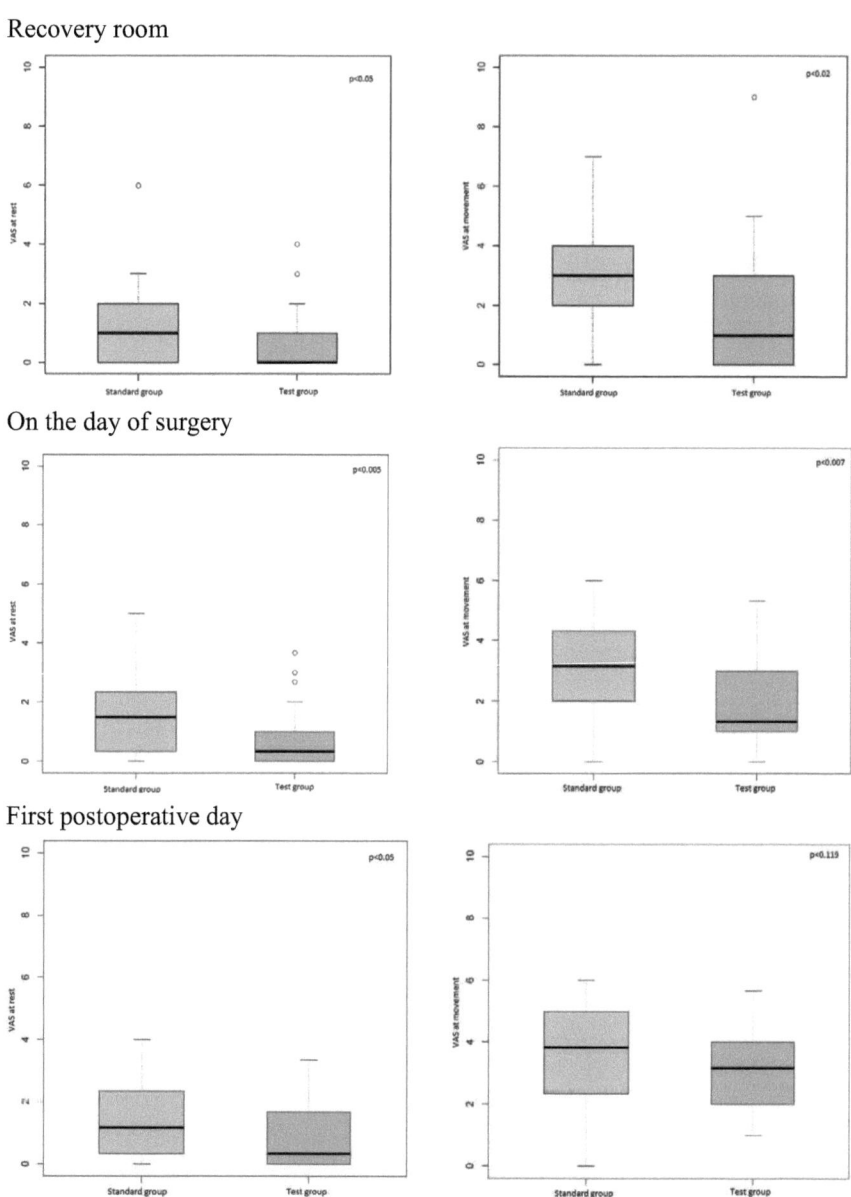

Graph 1: VAS at rest (left) and on movement (right) in the recovery room, on the day of surgery and on the first postoperative day (first group of examinees – after axillary dissection)

4.1.2 Patients after Immediate Reconstruction with a Tissue Expander

Graph 2 shows pain intensity after immediate reconstruction according to the VAS scale measured in the recovery room, on the day of surgery and on the first postoperative day. Data on postoperative pain is presented in Table 6.

Table 6: Pain intensity (second group of examinees – after immediate reconstruction)

Pain		Group with a local anaesthetic*	Standard group*	Value p
VAS in the recovery room	on movement	3.0 (0-8)	4.0 (1-9)	0.03
	at rest	3.0 (1-8)	5.0 (1-10)	0.01
VAS on the day of surgery	on movement	1.9 (0.2-4.8)	2.1 (0-8.8)	0.23
	at rest	3.8 (1.2-7.8)	4.8 (1.2-10)	0.003
VAS first postoperative day	on movement	1.5 (0-4.7)	1.7 (0-8)	0.69
	at rest	4.0 (0.7-6)	3.7 (0.7-9)	0.96
Pain after three months (*number of patients*)		5 (17 %)	15 (50 %)	0.01

*Numerical variables in the parentheses are listed as an average value (SD) or median (range); for descriptive variables, numbers are listed (%). The data which is not in the parentheses is listed as VAS values.

Recovery room

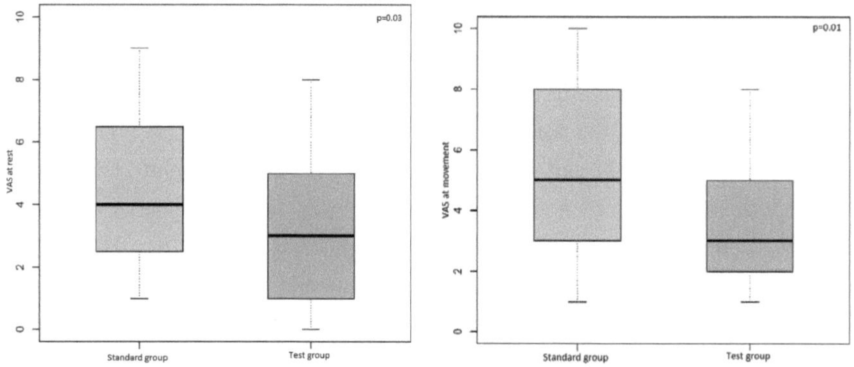

On the day of surgery

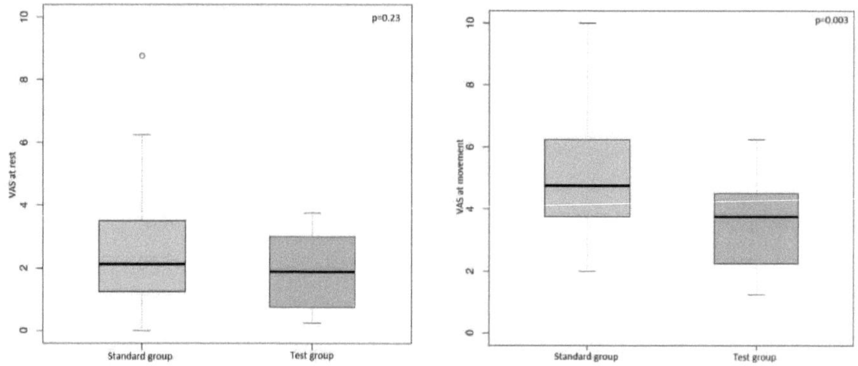

First postoperative day

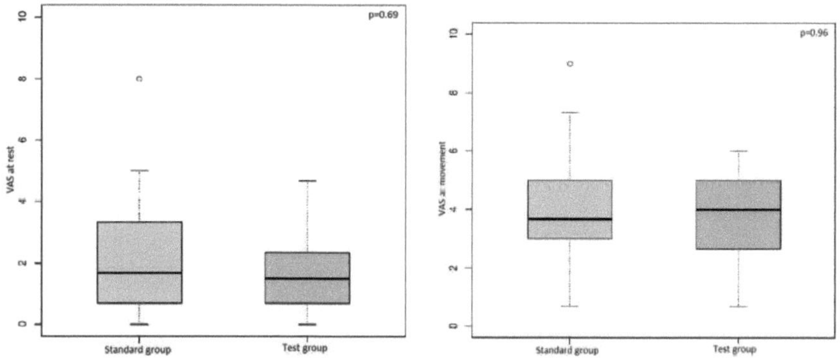

Graph 2: VAS at rest (left) and on movement (right) in the recovery room, on the day of surgery and on the first postoperative day (second group of examinees – after immediate reconstruction)

4.1 Consumption of Opioids and Other Analgesics, Alertness

Piritramide consumption in the first 24 hours postoperatively was lower in the test group in comparison to the control group, both after axillary lymph node dissection ($p < 0.0001$) (Graph 3) and immediate reconstruction ($p < 0.0001$). Metamizole consumption in the first 24 hours postoperatively was also significantly lower in the test group with the local anaesthetic in both groups of examinees ($p < 0.0001$). There were no differences between the test and the standard group in both groups of examinees regarding the consumption of diclofenac – analgesic tablets. But the consumption of tablets of paracetamole with tramadol was lower ($p = 0,035$) in the test group of the first group of examinees (axillary dissection patients), thought there were no differences in consumption between the test and the standard group of the second group of examinees (immediate reconstruction patients). Alertness measured 6 hours postoperatively was higher in the test group in comparison to the control group in both groups of examinees (after axillary node dissection $p = 0.001$; after immediate reconstruction $p < 0.001$). Data on drug consumption and alertness for the first group of examinees (axillary dissection patients) is presented in Table 7 and Graph 3 and 4 on the left side, and the data for the second group of examinees (immediate reconstruction patients) is presented in Table 8 and Graph 3 and 4 on the right side.

Table 7: Drug consumption and alertness (first group of examinees – after axillary dissection)

Drugs	Group with a local anaesthetic*	Standard group*	Value p
Piritramide – consumption in the first 24 hours (mg)	7.5 (7.5-10.5)	19.4 (7.5-37.5)	< 0.0001
Metamizole – consumption in the first 24 hours (g)	2.5 (0-5)	3.5 (0.5)	<0.0001
Metoclopramide - consumption in the first 24 hours (mg)	10 (0-10)	17.7 (6.7-30.1)	< 0.0001
Tramadol/paracetamole - consumption in the first three days (tablets)	4 (0-11)	6 (1-13)	0.035
Diclofenac - consumption in the first three days (mg)	200 (0-300)	200 (0-300)	0.13
Alertness OAA/S** six hours after surgery	5.0 (4-5)	4.5 (3-5)	0.001

*Numerical variables are listed as median (range);
**OAA/S - observer's assessment of alertness/sedation

Table 8: Drug consumption and alertness (second group of examinees – after immediate reconstruction)

Drugs	Group with a local anaesthetic*	Standard group*	Value p
Piritramide – consumption in the first 24 hours (mg)	7.5 (7.5-28.5)	28.4 (16.1-51.7)	< 0.0001
Metamizole – consumption in the first 24 hours (g)	2.5 (2.5-5)	4.1 (2.9-7.5)	< 0.0001
Metoclopramide - consumption in the first 24 hours (mg)	10.0 (10-30)	22.9 (10-40)	< 0.0001
Tramadol/paracetamole - consumption in the first four days (tablets)	19.0 (1-30)	18.0 (6-30)	0.46
Diclofenac - consumption in the first four days (mg)	400.0 (100-400)	400.0 (100-550)	0.57
Alertness OAA/S** six hours after surgery	5.0 (4-5)	5.0 (3-5)	< 0.001

*Numerical variables are listed as median (range);
**OAA/S - observer's assessment of alertness/sedation

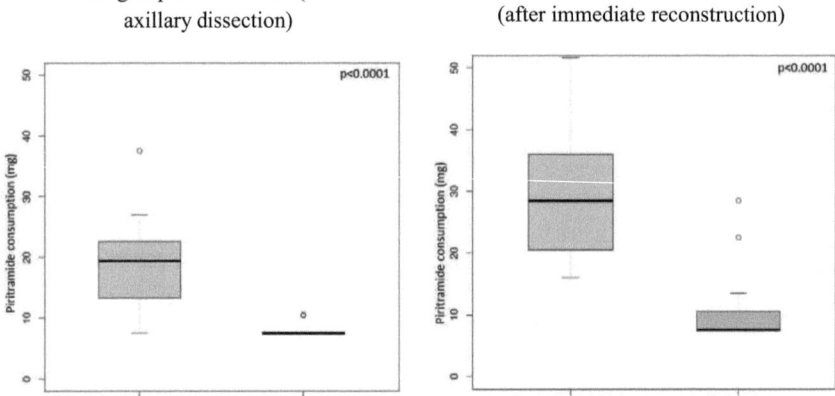

Graph 3: Piritramide consumption in the first 24 postoperative hours

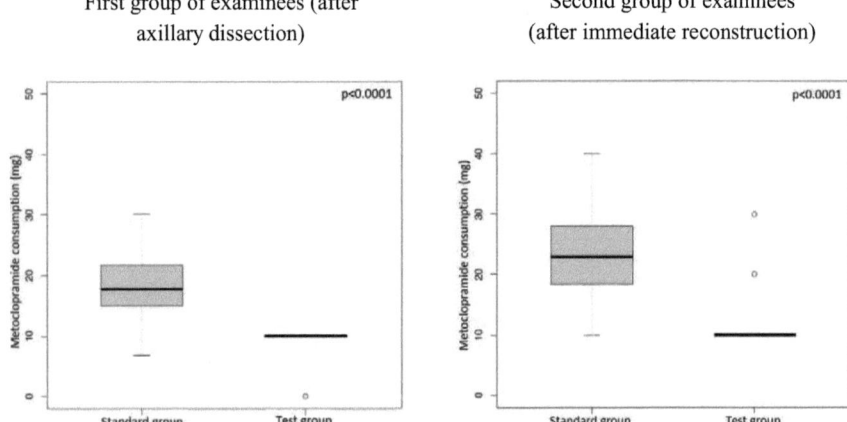

Graph 4: Metoclopramide consumption in the first 24 postoperative hours

4.1 Postoperative Nausea

Patients in the test group experienced less postoperative nausea than patients in the standard group, which is true for in both groups of examinees. Metoclopramide consumption in the first 24 hours postoperatively was lower in the test group than in the control standard group, which is true for both groups of examinees ($p < 0.0001$). Data on metoclopramide consumption after axillary dissection is presented in Table 7 and Graph 4 on the left side, data on metoclopramide consumption after immediate reconstruction is presented in Table 8 and Graph 4 on the right side.

4.2 Complications

No local signs of an infection were noticed in the area where the catheter was inserted in any of the patients. All collected microbiological samples were negative. There were no significant differences between the test group and the standard group, which is true for both groups of examinees. Inflammation resolved after treatment with antibiotics and the tissue expander remained in place. In the first group of examinees (axillary dissection patients), complications occurred in 15 patients (25 %). In the second group of examinees (immediate reconstruction patients), complications occurred in nine patients (15 %). Data on complications after operation after axillary lymph node dissection is presented in Table 3; data on complications after operation after immediate reconstruction is presented in Table 4.

4.3 Hospitalization

Average length of hospitalization in the first group of examinees (axillary dissection patients) was 1.7 days. There was no significant difference in the length of hospitalization between the standard group and the group with a local anaesthetic in the first group of examinees ($p = 0.22$). Average length of hospitalization in the second group of examinees (immediate reconstruction patients) was 5.3 days. There was no significant difference in the length of hospitalization between the standard group and the group with a local anaesthetic in the second group of examinees ($p = 0.61$). Data on length of hospitalization for both groups of examinees is presented in Table 3 and Table 4.

4.4 Late Complications

Three months after surgery, patients were asked about the presence of pain in the operated area. Fifteen patients (50 %) from the standard group who received intravenous analgesia reported that pain was still present after axillary dissection. In the test group with a local anaesthetic in the wound, however, only five patients (17 %) reported that pain was still present, which is significantly less ($p = 0.01$). The presence of pain three and six moths after axillary lymph node dissection is presented in Table 5.

The same result was obtained after immediate reconstruction. The presence of pain three and six moths after axillary lymph node dissection is presented in Table 6. The presence of pain after six month was not established in the second group of examinees (after immediate reconstruction), because at that time, the patients were again undergoing surgery for permanent implant insertion. Patients after immediate reconstruction were asked about swelling of the upper limb three months postoperatively. Lymphedema was reported by two patients after immediate breast reconstruction, one patient from the test group who underwent axillary dissection during the operation and one patient from the standard group who underwent bilateral sentinel node biopsy.

Patients answered a questionnaire on neuropathic pain six months after axillary lymph node dissection.[2] We assessed the presence of reduced arm mobility and the presence of lymphedema. 18 patients (30 %) experienced chronic neuropathic pain, 6 patients (20 %) from the test group with a local anaesthetic and 12 patients from the standard group (40 %) (p = 0.09). Lymphedema of the upper limb was present in 21 patients, in 10 patients from the standard group and 11 patients from the test group with a local anaesthetic. Restricted mobility was present in 14 patients (23.3 %), 7 from each group. There were no differences in frequency of chronic pain between the test and the standard group after adjuvant treatment – Table 5.

5 DISCUSSION

Axillary lymph node dissection is the standard surgical procedure in breast cancer or melanoma in case of metastases in the lymph nodes (59-61). Axillary lymph node dissection is connected with long-term consequences: chronic postoperative pain, restrained shoulder mobility and/or lymphedema (17-19). Severe postoperative pain is characteristic after subpectoral breast augmentation and after breast reconstruction with a tissue expander (17,24,47-50,53,54). Legeby *et al.* established that pain is much more severe three hours after immediate reconstruction with a tissue expander than after mastectomy or axillary dissection (17). The average VAS score during the

---

[2] The questionnaire on neuropatic pain is a standardized international form - DN4. We use the Slovene version of the questionnaire, listed under Appendix 1 in this study, at the Institute of Oncology.

first three hours after immediate breast reconstruction was 4.9 or 5 in simultaneous axillary dissection. The average VAS score during the first three hours after mastectomy was only 2.1 and 3 after mastectomy with axillary dissection (17). Similar results were observed also in our study after immediate breast reconstruction with a tissue expander, as patients reported a VAS score that was 3 units higher on average in the recovery room than after axillary dissection without reconstruction (62). The average VAS score in the recovery room after reconstruction was 4.9 in the standard group and 3.4 in the group with a local anaesthetic. The average VAS score in the recovery room after axillary dissection was 2 in the standard group and 0.5 in the group with a local anaesthetic. The local anaesthetic reduced pain for 1.5 VAS units more than standard treatment in both groups of examinees. Based on the above stated we conclude that immediate breast reconstruction with a tissue expander is connected with more than one time more severe postoperative acute pain than after axillary lymph node dissection.

The most encouraging result of our study found in the second group of examinees (immediate reconstruction patients) is that as much as 77 % of the patients did not experience severe pain immediately after the operation. As far as we know, there are no reports in literature on similarly effective postoperative analgesia after insertion of a tissue expander. Legeby *et al.* reported the occurrence of unexpected severe pain in as much as 48 % in patients treated with a local anaesthetic (VAS 4.7 – 10) (17). Legeby used an epidural catheter that had only a few perforations and the local anaesthetic was applied every three hours. We used the continuous method of application of a local anaesthetic and a catheter with numerous perforations 15 cm in length. In our opinion, this is the reason why only 7 patients had a VAS score higher than 5 (23 %), while there were 13 such patients in the control group (42 %). Efficacy of analgesia with a local anaesthetic was noticeable on the day of surgery, significant difference in pain intensity between the groups no longer existed in the following days. But pain is already bearable by then and manageable mostly by oral analgesics. Consumption of a combination of tramadol and paracetamol tablets in patients after axillary dissection during hospitalization was lower in the test group compared to the standard group (p = 0.035). There were no differences between the two groups of patients after reconstruction in consumption of tablets with a combination of tramadol and paracetamol, which is understandable, because the operation is much more painful.

Our study has shown that continuous infusion of a local anaesthetic into the surgical wound reduces pain after breast surgery and at the same time reduces opioid consumption – pritramide, similarly as the majority of other studies on the significance of local anaesthetics for postoperative pain treatment have shown (13,19,24,31,53,54). Reduced piritramide consumption was present in the patient group with local anaesthetics both after axillary lymph node dissection and after immediate reconstruction. Legeby *et al.* discovered that opioid consumption in the first three hours after immediate reconstruction is three times higher than after other breast cancer operations. Opioid consumption after insertion of a tissue expander was 11.8 mg or 12.8 mg with simultaneous axillary dissection, while opioid consumption after mastectomy was 3.2 mg or 5.5 mg with simultaneous axillary dissection (17). Our patients with standard analgesia required 5.6-times more opioids after insertion of a tissue expander during the first three postoperative hours than patients after axillary lymph node dissection (62). Pain intensity was strongest during the first three postoperative days. Opioid consumption in the first 24 hours was around three times lower in the group with a local anaesthetic than in the standard group, which is true for both groups of examinees. Consequently, patients in the group with a local anaesthetic with lower opioid consumption were less nauseas, which can be seen in lower metoclopramide consumption in the test group. This is true for both groups of examinees.

The second very important aim of treating breast cancer patients after axillary lymph node dissection is the occurrence of chronic pain. Axillary lymph node dissection causes chronic problems in the sense of neuropathic pain, arm swelling and reduced arm functionality. Effective postoperative pain treatment is important, because it can prevent the occurrence of chronic pain (2). Many factors are involved in the development of chronic postoperative pain: genetic predisposition, psychosocial background, age and gender (5). Smith *et al.* found the following risk factors for the development of a post mastectomy pain syndrome: age, marital status, employment status and housing (63). Many studies have proven that severe postoperative pain is connected with the development of chronic postoperative pain (64). Thusly, it has been proven that infusion of a local anaesthetic into the peripheral nerve pericyte reduces the occurrence of chronic pain after lower limb amputation (65). An epidural block before surgery reduces long-term post-thoracotomy pain (66).

The use of local anaesthetics immediately after surgery with the purpose of reducing the occurrence of post-mastectomy syndrome has not been sufficiently researched so far. Three months after axillary lymph node dissection, our patients who were treated with continuous infusion of a local anaesthetic into the wound reported less frequently that pain was still present than the group with standard treatment (17 % vs. 50 %; p = 0.01). Six months after axillary lymph node dissection, only a trend towards reduced pain was still noticeable in the group with continuous infusion of a local anaesthetic in the wound in comparison with opioid analgesia (20 % vs. 40 %; p = 0.09). Fassoulaki et al. reported similar results regarding the presence of post-mastectomy syndrome (31,45). In the first study, where a crème with a local anaesthetic was used, chronic pain was present in 43 % after three months, and as much as in 91 % in the control group (p = 0.002). In the second study, in which the multimodal approach was used, pain was present in 45 % after three months, and in 82 % in the control group (p = 0.028). After six months, only a trend towards reduced chronic pain was still present in the test group 30 % : 57 %, which was no longer statistically significant. It is obvious that a local anaesthetic used during operation can affect the frequency and intensity of pain in the subcutaneous phase. But the question is whether it can affect the occurrence of post mastectomy syndrome. In our study, we did not notice differences in arm swelling or the upper limb mobility in the shoulder in our patients. Occurrence of pain was reduced after the use of a local anaesthetic. But well-treated acute pain enables good rehabilitation and arm exercise immediately after surgery. In order to prove the effect of intensive exercise after axillary lymph node dissection, additional prospective studies are necessary.

A reduced occurrence of chronic pain was recorded in the test group three months after surgery also in patients after immediate reconstruction. Only five patients (17 %) from the group with a local anaesthetic and as much as 15 patients from the standard group (50 %) (p = 0.01) reported that pain was still present, which is completely the same as in patients after axillary dissection. After six months, most patients again underwent surgery for implant insertion, which is why the presence of chronic pain was not established after six months.

An analysis of the costs of treatment was not performed. The costs of drugs in the test group and the standard group were practically the same, because prices of intravenous drugs and tablets are low. Treatment with an elastomeric pump is 175

EUR more expensive than standard treatment, which is the price of an elastomeric pump and a perforated catheter. But we have proven that patients treated with continuous infusion of a local anaesthetic into the wound are more alert than patients who received standard treatment with an intravenous opioid. Almost all of the patients treated with a local anaesthetic had a high alertness score according OAA/S already on the day of surgery. In our opinion, this could enable discharge from hospital already on the day of surgery in patients after axillary lymph node dissection, which is already the practice in some hospitals, e.g. in the Memorial Sloan-Kettering Cancer Centre in New York. Hospitalization after immediate reconstruction could also be shortened considering the reduced pain after continuous infusion of a local anaesthetic. Surgery without pain and shorter hospitalization are the foundation of a patient-friendly treatment.

There were no differences in complications, as are haemorrhage, inflammation or hemodynamic instability, between the two groups, which was established also by other authors who studied the significance of analgesia with local anaesthetics (13,19,24,44-54,67-71). Contrary to this, some authors reported a reduced occurrence of inflammation with the use of local anaesthetics (72,73,74). Just as other authors, we did not record any toxic adverse effects of local anaesthetics. In our study, we used 0.25 % levobupivacaine, which is listed as one of the safer local anaesthetics (57).

In our study, we confirmed the efficacy of 0.25 % levobupivacaine, a local anaesthetic, in the surgical wound for the treatment of acute postoperative pain and a reduced occurrence of chronic pain after three months. We have confirmed that treatment with a local anaesthetic is more effective and has less adverse effects in comparison to treatment with intravenous opioids. Patients were more alert after surgery as after standard treatment with intravenous opioids. Patients were less nauseous postoperatively, they required less antiemetics than the standard group.

Pain after surgery is greater if the patient feels anxious (15). In our opinion, the patients would be better prepared for treatment, if they were well informed about the methods of treatment. Including nurses in the process of informing patients has proven itself as a very important factor of satisfaction and good clinical practice (75).

6 CONCLUSIONS

Our study was conducted on two groups of examinees: the first group of examinees comprised patients after axillary lymph node dissection, the second group comprised patients after immediate reconstruction with a tissue expander. Both groups were randomized into the test group with 0.25 % levobupivacaine, a local anaesthetic, in the surgical wound and the standard group with continuous intravenous analgesia.

With the doctor's thesis and study related to it we have confirmed the working hypothesis that patients treated only with local anaesthetics applied to the wound by catheter with a self-deflating pump have less pain than patients treated only with systemic analgesics.

All the specific aims of the study were confirmed:

1. Patients treated with a local anaesthetic have less pain after axillary dissection for breast cancer than patients treated only with systemic analgesics.
2. Patients treated with a local anaesthetic have less pain after immediate breast reconstruction with a tissue expander than patients treated only with systemic analgesics.
3. Patients treated with a local anaesthetic require less opioids and antiemetics and are more alert after axillary dissection for breast cancer than patients treated only with systemic analgesics.
4. Patients treated with a local anaesthetic require less opioids and antiemetics and are more alert after immediate breast reconstruction with a tissue expander than patients treated only with systemic analgesics.
5. Chronic pain after axillary dissection for breast cancer occurs less frequently in patients treated with a local anaesthetic than in patients treated only with systemic analgesics.
6. Chronic pain after immediate breast reconstruction with a tissue expander occurs less frequently in patients treated with a local anaesthetic than in patients treated only with systemic analgesics.

7 SOURCES AND LITERATURE

1. IASP. International Association for the Study of Pain. [Online].; 2013 [accessed 24.5.2013]. Access on: http://www.iasp-pain.org/AM/Template.cfm?Section=Pain_Definitions .
2. Kehlet H. Postoperative pain relief-what is the issue? Br J Anaesth 1994; 72(4):375-8.
3. Biki B, Mascha E, Moriarty D, Fitzpatrick JM, Sessler DI, Buggy D. Anesthetic Technique for Radical Prostatectomy Surgery Affects Cancer Recurrence: A Retrospective Analysis. Anesthesiology 2008; 109(2):180-7.
4. Werner MU, Søholm L, Rotbøll-Nielsen P, Kehlet H. Does an Acute Pain Service Improve Postoperative Outcome? Anesth Analg 2002; 95(5):1361-72.
5. Kehlet H, Jensen TS, Woolf CJ. Persistent postsurgical pain: risk factors and prevention. The Lancet 2006; 367(9522):1618-25.
6. Rubinson K, Lang EJ. The nervous system. V Koeppen B, Stanton B. Berne&Levy: Physiology. 6th ed.: Elsevier; 2010. str. 53-230.
7. Almeida TF, Roizenblatt S, Tufik S. Afferent pain pathways: a neuroanatomical review. Brain Research 2004; 1000(1-2):40-56.
8. Hall JE. Guyton and Hall Textbook of Medical Physiology. 12th ed.: Saunders; 2011.
9. Campbell WW. DeJongs The Neurologic Examination. 7th ed.: DeJong; 2012.
10. Jones HR, Burns TM, Aminhoff MJ, Pomeroy SL. The Netter Collection of Medical Illustrations:Nervous System: Part II Spinal Cord and Peripheral Motor and Sensory Systems. 2nd ed.: Elsevier Science; 2013.
11. Zhang YQ. The Affective Dimension of Pain. V Lucas , Alexandre , uredniki. Frontiers in Pain Research. 1st ed.: Nova Science Pub Inc; 2006. str. 28-47.
12. Moore KL, Agur AMR, Dalley AF. Clinically oriented anatomy. 6th ed.: Lippincott Williams & Wilkins; 2010.
13. Jacobs VR, Morrison JE. Application of a locally placed anesthesia catheter for reduction of postoperative pain after mastectomy for breast cancer. Int J Fertil Women's Med 2006; 51(5):225-9.
14. Merskey H, Bogduk N. Classification of chronic pain: Descriptions of chronic pain syndromes and definitions of pain terms. 2nd ed. Seattle: IASP Press; 1994.

15. Katz J, Poleshuck EL, Andrus CH, Hogan LA, Jung BF, Kulick DI, et al. Risk factors for acute pain and its persistence following breast cancer surgery. Pain 2005; 119(1-3):16-25.

16. Gedney JJ, Logan H. Pain related recall predicts future pain report. Pain 2006; 121(1):69-76.

17. Legeby M, Segerdahl M, Sandelin K, Wickman M, Ostman K, Olofsson CH. Immediate reconstruction in breast cancer surgery requires intensive post-operative pain treatment but the effects of axillary dissection may be more predictive of chronic pain. Breast 2002; 11(2):156-62.

18. Lahajnar-Čavlović S. Bolečina po operaciji raka dojk: Rezultati raziskave med bolnicami na Onkološkem inštitutu v Ljubljani. Onkologija 2007; 9(2):114-8.

19. Schell SR. Patient outcomes after axillary lymph node dissection for breast cancer: use of postoperative continuous local anesthesia infusion. J Surg Res 2006; 134(1):124-32.

20. Tasmuth T, Kataja M, Blomqvist Cl, Von Smittent Kl, Kalso E. Treatment-Related Factors Predisposing to Chronic Pain in Patients with Breast Cancer. Acta Onclogica 1997; 36(6):625-30.

21. Lubenow TR, Ivankovich AD, McCarthy RJ. Management of acute postoperative pain. V Barash PG, Culler BF, Stoelting RK. Clinical Anesthesia.: JB Lippincott Company; 1995. str. 1547-77.

22. Garcia-Etienne CA, Forcellini D, Sagona A, Caviggioli F, Barbieri E, Cornegliani G, et al. Breast reconstruction: a quality measure for breast cancer care? Breast 2012; 21(1):105-6.

23. Spear SL, Spittler CJ. Breast reconstruction with implants and expanders. Plast Reconstr Surg 2001; 107(1):177-87.

24. Rawal N, Gupta A, Helsing M, Grell K, Allvin R. Pain relief following breast augmentation surgery: a comparison between incisional patient-controlled regional analgesia and traditional oral analgesia. Eur J Anaesthesiol 2006; 23(12):1010-7.

25. Marchettini P, Simone DA, Caputi G, Ochoa JL. Pain from excitation of identified muscle nociceptors in humans. Brain Researc 1996; 740(1-2):109-16.

Appendix 1: DN4 Questionnaire

DN4 – QUESTIONNAIRE

To estimate the probability of neuropathic pain, please answer yes or no for each item of the following four questions.

INTERVIEW OF THE PATIENT

QUESTION 1:
Does the pain have one or more of the following characteristics?	YES	NO
Burning	☐	☐
Painful cold	☐	☐
Electric shocks	☐	☐

QUESTION 2:
Is the pain associated with one or more of the following symptoms in the same area?	YES	NO
Tingling	☐	☐
Pins and needles	☐	☐
Numbness	☐	☐
Itching	☐	☐

EXAMINATION OF THE PATIENT

QUESTION 3:
Is the pain located in an area where the physical examination may reveal one or more of the following characteristics?	YES	NO
Hypoesthesia to touch	☐	☐
Hypoesthesia to pinprick	☐	☐

QUESTION 4:
In the painful area, can the pain be caused or increased by:	YES	NO
Brushing?	☐	☐

YES = 1 point
NO = 0 points

Patient's Score: /10

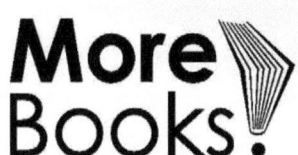
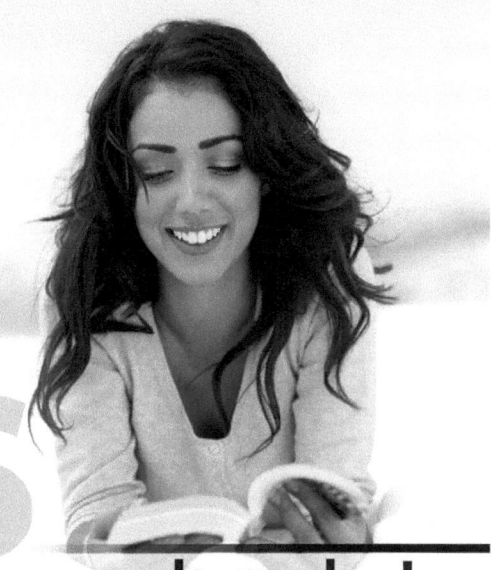

I want morebooks!

Buy your books fast and straightforward online - at one of the world's fastest growing online book stores! Environmentally sound due to Print-on-Demand technologies.

Buy your books online at
www.get-morebooks.com

Kaufen Sie Ihre Bücher schnell und unkompliziert online – auf einer der am schnellsten wachsenden Buchhandelsplattformen weltweit! Dank Print-On-Demand umwelt- und ressourcenschonend produziert.

Bücher schneller online kaufen
www.morebooks.de

OmniScriptum Marketing DEU GmbH
Heinrich-Böcking-Str. 6-8
D - 66121 Saarbrücken
Telefax: +49 681 93 81 567-9

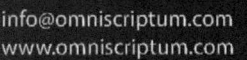
info@omniscriptum.com
www.omniscriptum.com

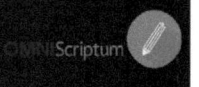

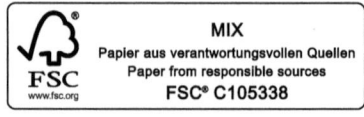

Printed by Books on Demand GmbH, Norderstedt / Germany